FAST FACTS

Long-Chain Fatty Acid Oxidation Disorders

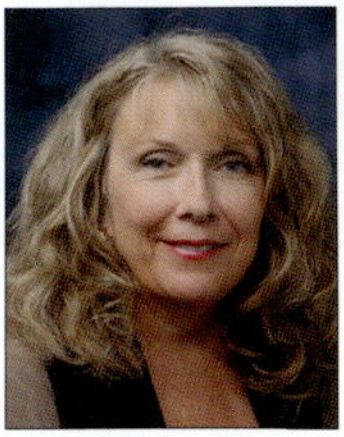

Barbara K Burton MD
Professor of Pediatrics
(Genetics, Birth Defects, and Metabolism)
Ann & Robert H Lurie Children's Hospital of Chicago
Chicago, Illinois
USA

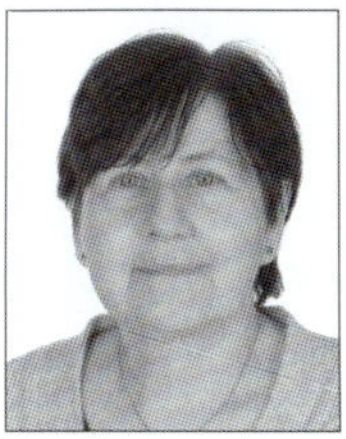

Anne Daly MSc
Specialist Metabolic Dietitian
Departments of Dietetics and
Inherited Metabolic Disorders
Birmingham Children's Hospital
Birmingham, UK

Declaration of Independence

This book is as balanced and as practical as we can make it.
Ideas for improvement are always welcome: fastfacts@karger.com

KARGER

Fast Facts: Long-Chain Fatty Acid Oxidation Disorders
First published 2021

S. Karger Publishers Ltd, Elizabeth House, Queen Street,
Abingdon, Oxford OX14 3LN, UK; Tel: +44 (0)1235 523233

Book orders can be placed by telephone or email, or via the website.
Please telephone +41 61 306 1440 or email orders@karger.com
To order via the website, please go to karger.com

A CIP record for this title is available from the British Library.

ISBN 978-3-318-06830-6

Burton B (Barbara)
Fast Facts: Long-Chain Fatty Acid Oxidation Disorders/
Barbara K Burton, Anne Daly

Typesetting by Amnet, Chennai, India.
Printed in the UK with Xpedient Print.

Cover image: a colored transmission electron micrograph (TEM) of a mitochondrion inside a cell. K.R. Porter/Science Photo Library

An independent publication developed by S. Karger Publishers Limited and provided as a service to medicine. Supported by an educational grant from Ultragenyx Pharmaceutical Inc.

List of abbreviations and glossary

ACAD9: acyl-CoA dehydrogenase family, member 9

***ACADM*:** gene encoding medium-chain acyl-CoA dehydrogenase

***ACADVL*:** gene encoding very-long-chain acyl-CoA dehydrogenase

C0: free carnitine

CACT: carnitine–acylcarnitine translocase

CK: creatine kinase

CoA: coenzyme A

CPT1: carnitine palmitoyltransferase 1. There are different isoforms: a liver isoform (CPT1-L), encoded by *CPT1A*; a muscle and heart isoform (CPT1-M), encoded by *CPT1B*; and a brain isoform (CPT1-B), encoded by *CPT1C*. These isoforms have different kinetic properties. A mutation associated with a fatty acid oxidation disorder has been identified only in *CPT1A* in humans, and the defect is generally referred to as CPT1 deficiency

CPT2: carnitine palmitoyltransferase 2

CTD: carnitine transporter deficiency

CUD: carnitine uptake defect, an alternative name for carnitine transporter deficiency

***ETFA*:** gene encoding electron transfer flavoprotein subunit α

***ETFB*:** gene encoding electron transfer flavoprotein subunit β

***ETFDH*:** gene encoding electron transfer flavoprotein dehydrogenase

FAD: flavin adenine dinucleotide

$FADH_2$: reduced form of FAD

FAOD: fatty acid oxidation disorder

HAD: 3-hydroxyacyl-CoA dehydrogenase

***HADH*:** gene encoding 3-hydroxyacyl-CoA dehydrogenase

***HADHA*:** gene encoding 3-hydroxyacyl-CoA dehydrogenase trifunctional multienzyme complex subunit α

***HADHB*:** gene encoding 3-hydroxyacyl-CoA dehydrogenase trifunctional multienzyme complex subunit β

HELLP: hemolysis, elevated liver enzymes and low platelets (syndrome)

HMG: 3-hydroxy-3-methylglutaryl

HSL: hormone-sensitive lipase

LC: long-chain

LCEH: long-chain-enoyl-CoA hydratase

LCFA: long-chain fatty acid

LCHAD: long-chain 3-hydroxyacyl-CoA dehydrogenase

LCKAT: long-chain 3-ketoacyl-CoA thiolase

MADD: multiple acyl-CoA dehydrogenase deficiency, also known as glutaric aciduria type 2 (GA2)

MCAD: medium-chain acyl-CoA dehydrogenase

MCFA: medium-chain fatty acid

MTP: mitochondrial trifunctional protein (also known as trifunctional protein [TFP])

NAD: nicotinamide adenine dinucleotide

NADH: reduced form of NAD

NEFA: non-esterified fatty acid (also known as free fatty acid)

OCTN2: organic cation/carnitine transporter 2 (also known as SLC22A5 [solute carrier family 22 member 5])

SCAD: short-chain acyl-CoA dehydrogenase

SCHAD: short-chain 3-hydroxyacyl-CoA dehydrogenase

SCFA: short-chain fatty acid

***TANGO2*:** gene encoding transport and golgi organization 2 homolog

TFP: trifunctional protein (also known as mitochondrial trifunctional protein [MTP])

VLCAD: very-long-chain acyl-CoA dehydrogenase

VLFA: very-long-chain fatty acid

Introduction

Disorders affecting the oxidation of long-chain fatty acids are complex, potentially life-threatening, metabolic conditions. A number of genetically distinct conditions exist, depending on the gene and protein affected, but there are some common clinical and biochemical features.

Newborn screening, which allows early intervention to prevent long-term morbidity, is not universally available. Even with screening, it is important that health professionals recognize the symptoms that may manifest at different stages of life.

This concise guide to these rare conditions will be of value to all health professionals who may encounter or care for an individual with a long-chain fatty acid oxidation disorder. As well as explaining the underlying defects, inheritance and how the conditions manifest, the book describes the diagnosis and differential diagnosis of the disorders. The final chapter gives some guidance on genetic counseling and supporting patients.

Each chapter is supported by key learning points, and we encourage you to take the free online FastTest that accompanies this resource at fastfacts.com to assess your understanding of these conditions.

We hope that this first edition of *Fast Facts: Long-Chain Fatty Acid Oxidation Disorders* will be a useful resource for anyone who has an interest in learning more about these genetic disorders of lipid metabolism.

1 Fatty acid metabolism

The term fatty acid oxidation refers to the breakdown of fatty acids, which are essential for the production of cellular energy. Fatty acids are a major fuel supplying energy during fasting and aerobic exercise. They serve most cells, with the exception of brain and red blood cells, and are the preferred respiratory fuel used by the heart and skeletal muscle, particularly during exercise. Oxidation of fatty acids during fasting provides up to 80% of total energy requirements.

Fatty acids

Fatty acids are carboxylic acids. In carboxylic acids, a carboxyl group (COOH) is attached to a second chemical group, referred to as R. In a fatty acid, R is a hydrocarbon chain (Figure 1.1).

Fatty acids have some general characteristics.

- The carbon chain length can vary between 4 and 28 units.
- The carbon chain can be saturated or unsaturated, branched or unbranched; most fatty acids have unbranched chains with an even number of carbon atoms.
- They are hydrophobic and are transported in the blood bound to albumin.
- They are characterized by their chain length:
  - short-chain fatty acids (SCFAs), with fewer than six carbons in the chain
  - medium-chain fatty acids (MCFAs), with six to 12 carbons

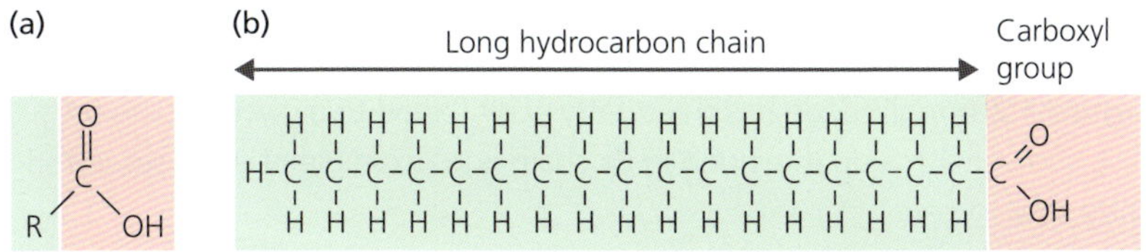

Figure 1.1 (a) The general structure of a carboxylic acid. (b) A fatty acid with a long hydrocarbon chain.

- long-chain fatty acids (LCFAs), with 13–21 carbons
- very-long-chain fatty acids (VLFAs), with 22 or more carbons.

Triglycerides

Fatty acids are consumed in the form of dietary triglycerides (sometimes called triacylglycerols), and adipocytes store triglycerides in large lipid droplets. Triglycerides form via a series of esterification reactions that link the carboxyl groups of three fatty acids to a glycerol backbone (Figure 1.2).

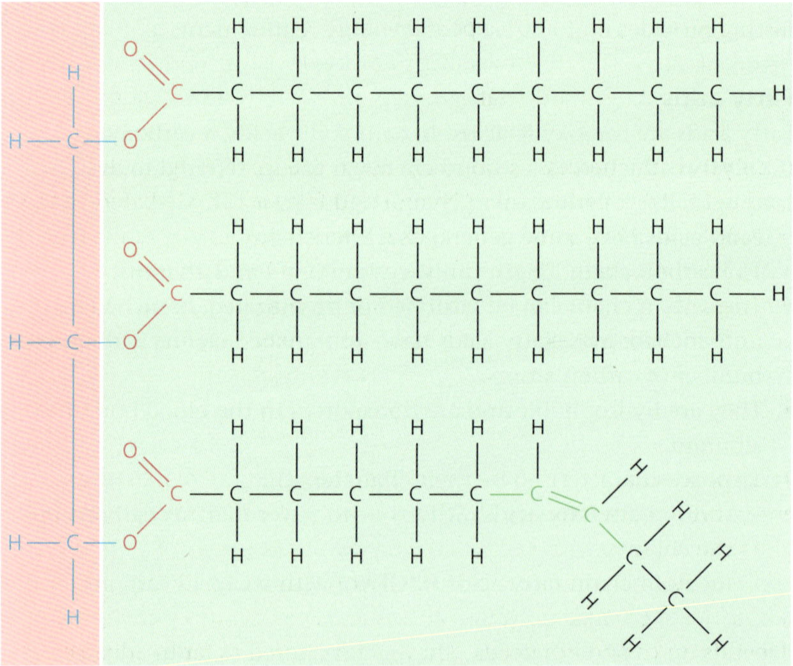

Figure 1.2 A triglyceride has three fatty acids joined to a glycerol. The fatty acid shown with a double bond in its chain is an example of an unsaturated fatty acid.

Absorption, transport and uptake of dietary fat

Absorption of fat occurs in three stages: emulsification, lipolysis and transportation. As fats are not naturally water soluble, they undergo several transformations before they can be utilized and transported around the body.

Emulsification is the formation of a homogeneous solution of two substances that are naturally immiscible (such as oil and water). Lipid (fat) globules containing triglycerides are emulsified in the intestine, a largely water-based environment. Bile salts, which are made in the liver, have an important role. They are amphipathic molecules, having both hydrophilic and hydrophobic portions. The hydrophilic portion is water soluble and the hydrophobic portion is fat soluble. The amphipathic nature of bile salts means they can emulsify the larger lipid globules to form smaller fat globules that can then undergo lipolysis (Figure 1.3).

Lipolysis is the process of breaking down the small fat globules containing triglycerides into glycerol and fatty acids. Mediated in the intestine mostly by pancreatic lipase, lipolysis involves a number of hydrolysis reactions. The result is a mixture of free fatty acids, monoglycerides and diglycerides, which then aggregate with bile salts and other amphipathic molecules to form mixed micelles. Micelles have a fatty core and a water-soluble outer lining and are easily absorbed by the intestinal enterocytes.

Transportation. Before fats can be absorbed into the bloodstream, the enterocytes reassemble free fatty acids and glycerol into triglycerides. These, together with cholesteryl ester, phospholipids and apolipoproteins, assemble to form chylomicrons, which then enter the bloodstream for transportation to tissues. The destiny of chylomicrons depends on the body's needs. They can be stored as fat in adipose tissue or undergo β-oxidation for energy. They are heterogeneous in size, composition and shape.

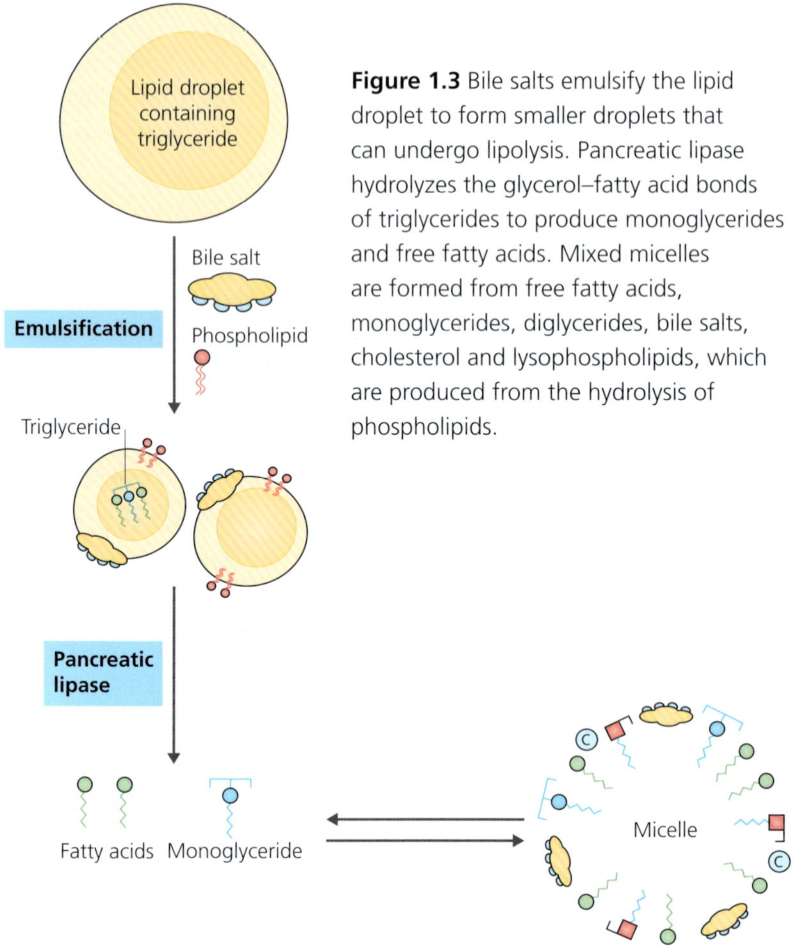

Figure 1.3 Bile salts emulsify the lipid droplet to form smaller droplets that can undergo lipolysis. Pancreatic lipase hydrolyzes the glycerol–fatty acid bonds of triglycerides to produce monoglycerides and free fatty acids. Mixed micelles are formed from free fatty acids, monoglycerides, diglycerides, bile salts, cholesterol and lysophospholipids, which are produced from the hydrolysis of phospholipids.

Fatty acid release from adipocytes is mediated by lipases, including hormone-sensitive lipase (HSL), which is under the control of hormones such as epinephrine (adrenaline) (Figure 1.4). Once released, the free fatty acids are transported, bound to albumin, in the blood and taken up by metabolizing cells.

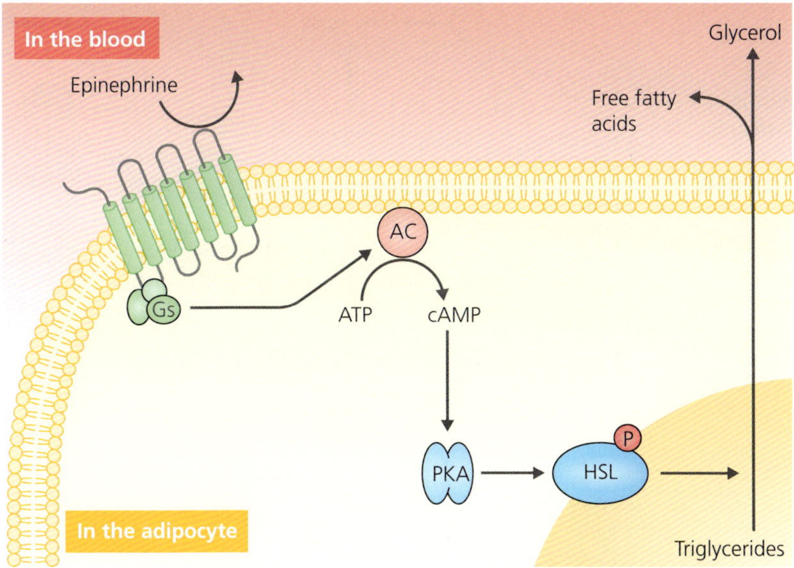

Figure 1.4 The interaction of epinephrine (adrenaline) with its receptor in the adipocyte cell membrane activates adenylyl cyclase (AC) via coupling to the trimeric G-protein, Gs. As a consequence, cyclic AMP (cAMP) is produced from ATP and activates AMP-dependent protein kinase A (PKA). PKA phosphorylates HSL, and the phosphorylated enzyme moves to the lipid droplet where, together with other lipases, it catalyzes the conversion of triglycerides to free fatty acids and glycerol.

Fatty acid breakdown

Fatty acid breakdown is an important reaction for energy production in a metabolizing cell. It involves several steps, controlled by hormones and enzymes (Figures 1.5 and 1.6). Deficiency of an enzyme involved in one of these steps results in a specific fatty acid oxidation disorder (FAOD).

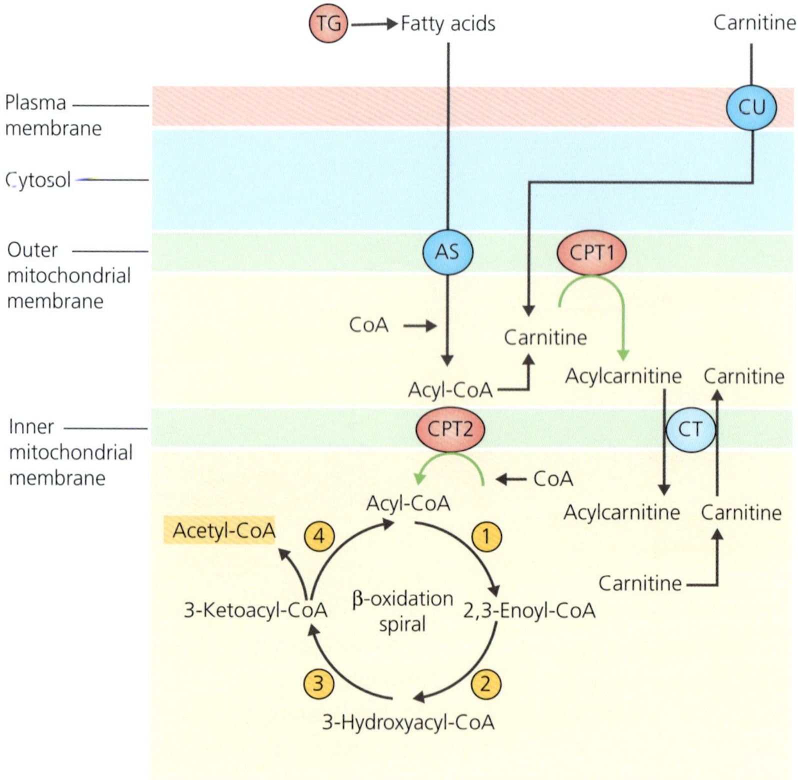

Figure 1.5 LCFAs are activated outside of the mitochondrial matrix to form acyl-CoAs in a reaction catalyzed by long-chain acyl-CoA synthetase or, for VLFAs, fatty acid transport protein (FATP) (shown in the figure as AS). As long-chain acyl-CoA molecules do not readily cross the inner mitochondrial membrane, the activated LCFAs are carried across by carnitine. Carnitine is accumulated inside cells by the high-affinity organic cation/carnitine transporter 2 (OCTN2) (shown as here as CU). Carnitine palmitoyltransferase (CPT) 1 catalyzes the formation of a high-energy bond between carnitine and LCFAs, and the resulting acylcarnitines are translocated across the inner mitochondrial membrane by carnitine–acylcarnitine translocase (CACT, shown here as CT). Inside the mitochondrion, CPT2, located in the inner mitochondrial membrane, removes carnitine from acylcarnitines and regenerates acyl-CoAs. The carnitine then returns to the cytoplasm and the LCFA undergoes rounds of β-oxidation within the mitochondrion. See Figure 1.6 for explanation of numbers 1–4. CoA, coenzyme A.

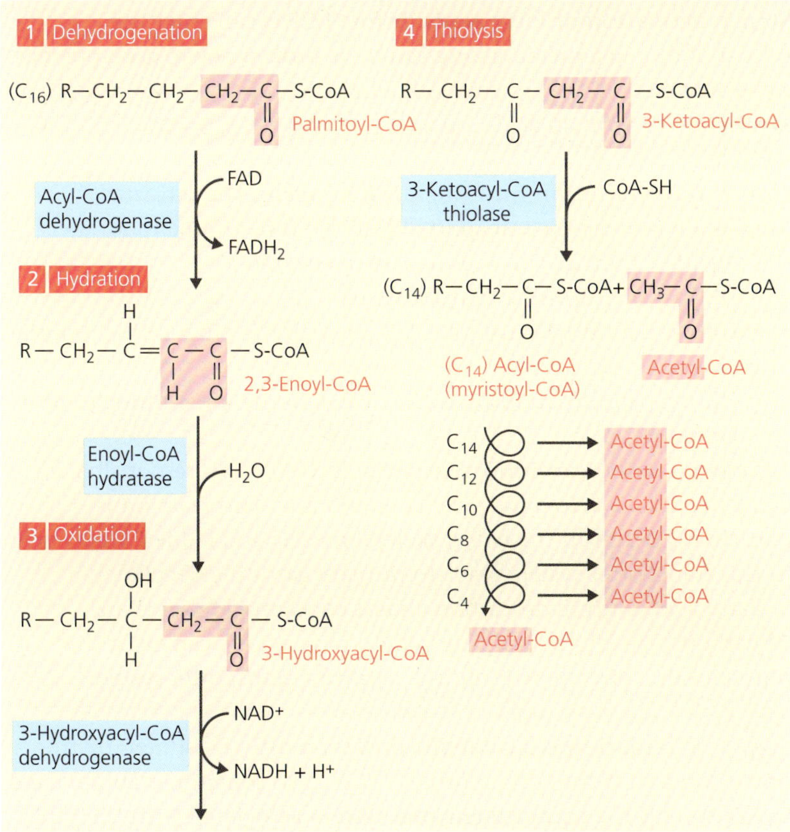

Figure 1.6 β-oxidation, shown here for palmitate (C16), comprises four steps. (1) Dehydrogenation: acyl-CoA is oxidized by acyl-CoA dehydrogenase, which is activated by flavin adenine dinucleotide (FAD), producing trans-enoyl-CoA. (2) Hydration: trans-enoyl-CoA is hydrated to produce 3-hydroxyacyl-CoA, catalyzed by 2,3-enoyl-CoA hydratase. (3) Oxidation: 3-hydroxyacyl-CoA oxidation is catalyzed by 3-hydroxyacyl-CoA dehydrogenase, activated by nicotinamide adenine dinucleotide (NAD), producing 3-ketoacyl-CoA. (4) Thiolysis: the 3-ketoacyl-CoA is split by a thiol group, catalyzed by 3-ketoacyl-CoA thiolase, producing acetyl-CoA and an acyl-CoA chain that is two carbon atoms shorter than when beginning the process.

Step 1: activation of fatty acids. Before LCFAs can enter the mitochondria of a metabolizing cell to be broken down, each one has to be activated by the enzyme long-chain acyl-coenzyme A (CoA) synthetase to form an acyl-CoA.

Step 2: transportation into the mitochondria. The activated long-chain acyl-CoA is transported into the inner mitochondria via the carnitine shuttle. This requires three enzymes:

- carnitine–acylcarnitine translocase (CACT)
- carnitine palmitoyltransferase 1 (CPT1), in the outer mitochondrial membrane
- carnitine palmitoyltransferase 2 (CPT2), in the inner mitochondrial membrane.

Organic cation/carnitine transporter 2 (OCTN2) is responsible for carnitine uptake across the plasma membrane. This reaction is particularly active in the heart, skeletal muscle and kidney. Deficiency in this transporter system leads to primary carnitine deficiency.

Fatty acids with hydrocarbon chains containing fewer than 12 carbons – medium- and short-chain fatty acids – can enter the mitochondria directly without the carnitine transporter system.

Step 3: β-oxidation is a catabolic process mostly facilitated by the mitochondrial trifunctional protein (TFP, also sometimes abbreviated to MTP). This is a complex enzyme system associated with the inner mitochondrial membrane. The TFP complex comprises two α subunits and two β subunits, encoded by *HADHA* and *HADHB*, respectively.

The α subunits function as two enzymes: long-chain-enoyl-CoA hydratase (LCEH) and long-chain 3-hydroxyacyl-CoA dehydrogenase (LCHAD).

The β subunits function as long-chain 3-ketoacyl-CoA thiolase (LCKAT).

Within the TFP complex, long straight-chain fatty acids are oxidized via a spiral pathway, with each turn in the pathway involving four enzyme reactions – dehydrogenation, hydration, oxidation and thiolysis – each catalyzed by a specific enzyme.

Step 4: the electron transport chain, also known as the respiratory chain, is embedded in the inner mitochondrial membrane. Electrons move from the reduced forms of both nicotinamide adenine dinucleotide (NAD) and flavin adenine dinucleotide (FAD) (NADH and $FADH_2$, respectively), which are produced during β-oxidation, through the transport chain to, ultimately, molecular oxygen. Energy released during the process establishes a proton gradient, which is used to generate ATP. Oxygen combines with hydrogen ions to form water.

Products. Each turn of the β-oxidation pathway involves removing two carbon atoms from the fatty acid chain, forming acetyl-CoA, NADH and $FADH_2$. Acetyl-CoA is used in the Krebs cycle or converted in the liver to produce ketone bodies via 3-hydroxy-3-methylglutaryl (HMG)-CoA synthase and lyase, while NADH and $FADH_2$ are passed to the electron transport chain. Both these pathways produce energy.

At the end of the oxidation process, acyl-CoA chains with an even number of carbon atoms are broken down to two acetyl-CoA units. Acyl-CoA chains with an odd number of carbons yield a five-carbon unit, which is broken down to a three-carbon propionyl-CoA and a two-carbon acetyl-CoA. The propionyl-CoA is then converted to succinyl-CoA, which enters the Krebs cycle to produce energy.

Disorders of fatty acid oxidation

Disruption at any point in the complex pathway described above leads to energy failure and characteristic clinical features. The biochemical hallmarks of these disorders are the accumulation of potentially toxic acylcarnitines, fatty acids and dicarboxylic acids in the urine and blood.

Key points – fatty acid metabolism

- Fatty acids are a major fuel supplying energy during fasting and aerobic exercise.
- Oxidation of fatty acids during fasting provides up to 80% of the body's total energy requirements.
- Fatty acids with a chain length of fewer than 12 carbons can enter mitochondria without the carnitine transporter carrier.
- Disruption at any point in the complex pathway of β-oxidation leads to energy failure and characteristic clinical features.

2 Epidemiology and genetics

FAODs are categorized as inborn errors of metabolism. They are a group of autosomal recessive inherited conditions present from birth. In countries offering newborn screening, FAODs are identified in the neonatal period. Where screening is not available, they may present at any time, often being precipitated during times of stress arising from illness, surgery, fasting or exercise.

There are a number of FAODs, and they are named depending on the specific defect or enzyme deficiency: for example, a short-, medium- or long-chain FAOD, or a transporter deficiency if the affected protein is involved in transporting fatty acids from one part of the cell to another (for example, carnitine transporter deficiency) (Table 2.1).

FAODs are primarily treated by dietary changes, which are disorder specific.

Incidence and prevalence

As a group, FAODs are among the most prevalent monogenic conditions worldwide; the combined incidence is estimated as 1:9300.[1] The prevalences of individual FAODs differ significantly (Table 2.2), and incidence can be difficult to estimate.

Very-long-chain acyl-CoA dehydrogenase (VLCAD) deficiency is the most common disorder of LCFA oxidation and its prevalence at birth has been estimated as 1:30 000 to 1:100 000.[2]

LCHAD deficiency/TFP deficiency is estimated to have a worldwide prevalence at birth of 1:250 000. It is known to be more common in some countries, such as Poland (1:120 000).[3]

FAODs have a particularly high incidence in populations of European origin, though certain FAODs have a higher frequency in some specific ethnic populations – CPT1 deficiency, for example, has a high frequency in the Inuit people of northern Canada.[4]

TABLE 2.1

Protein deficiencies causing fatty acid disorders

Deficiencies affecting the carnitine shuttle	
OCTN2	Organic cation/carnitine transporter 2 (carnitine transporter deficiency)
CPT1	Carnitine palmitoyltransferase 1
CACT	Carnitine–acylcarnitine translocase
CPT2	Carnitine palmitoyltransferase 2
Deficiencies affecting mitochondrial β-oxidation	
TFP/MTP	Mitochondrial trifunctional protein
VLCAD	Very-long-chain acyl-CoA dehydrogenase
LCHAD	Long-chain 3-hydroxyacyl-CoA dehydrogenase
MCAD	*Medium-chain acyl-CoA dehydrogenase*
SCAD	*Short-chain acyl-CoA dehydrogenase*
HMG-CoA	3-Hydroxy-3-methylglutaryl-CoA synthase/lyase
Other rare deficiencies affecting β-oxidation	
ACAD9	Acyl-CoA dehydrogenase family, member 9
*Crotonase**	*Short-chain enoyl-CoA hydratase*
HADH†	3-Hydroxyacyl-CoA dehydrogenase
DECR	2,4-Dienoyl-CoA reductase
Deficiencies affecting electon transfer	
MADD	*Multiple acyl-CoA dehydrogenase deficiency*

Those shown in italics are included for completeness but are outside of the scope of this book.
*Crotonase is also known as short-chain enoyl-CoA hydratase (SCEH or ECHS1).
†HADH deficiency is also known as M/SCHAD deficiency.

TABLE 2.2

Common genetic mutations in FAODs

Deficiency	Gene	Estimated prevalence of disorder	Common mutation
Disorders affecting the carnitine shuttle			
CPT1	*CPT1A*	1:500 000	Mild phenotype c.1436C>T Inuit, Alaskan Native
CACT	*CACT* (*SLC25A20*)	Rare	
CPT2	*CPT2*	Rare	c.338C>T (later-onset myopathic presentations)
CTD	*OCTN2* (*SLC22A5*)	1:20 000 to 1:120 000	
Disorders affecting mitochondrial β-oxidation			
VLCAD	*VLCAD* (*ACADVL*)	1:50 000 to 1:100 000	Mild or benign variant c.848T>C (also c.917T>C)
LCHAD	*HADHA*	1:110 000 to 1:150 000	c.1528G>C
TFP/MTP	*HADHA*, *HADHB*	Rare	
HADH	*HADH*	Rare	
Disorder affecting electron transfer			
MADD	*ETFA*, *ETFB*, *ETFDH*	Rare	

Where an older gene is shown, the up-to-date symbol is shown in parentheses. CTD, carnitine transporter deficiency; HAD, 3-hydroxyacyl-CoA dehydrogenase; MADD, multiple acyl-CoA dehydrogenase deficiency.

Impact of newborn screening programs. In countries with newborn screening programs, screening has led to the detection of many more affected infants than would have been predicted based on previous estimates of incidence.[2] Most individuals identified in this way are asymptomatic at the time of diagnosis.

Genetics

Inherited defects in 17 proteins directly affecting either carnitine-dependent transport or the process of β-oxidation have so far been identified.[5–8]

The phenotypes of FAODs are diverse, and they may be altered by genetic and environmental factors. Patients with medium-chain acyl-CoA dehydrogenase (MCAD) deficiency of the same genotype may die or remain asymptomatic, depending on their exposure to fasting stress. In contrast, the most common mutation associated with VLCAD deficiency in individuals of European descent, c.848T>C (p.Val283Ala), has been found only in mildly affected or asymptomatic patients. TFP deficiency, a clinically heterogeneous disorder with phenotypes of different severity, has been associated with a lethal mutation.[9]

The lack of a clear association between genotype and clinical symptoms makes clinical management particularly difficult. It is important to ensure patients have the optimal treatment to prevent possible clinical and life-threatening complications. Molecular heterogeneity has been described in all these fatty acid disorders, but some prevalent mutations have been identified (see Table 2.2).

Several mutations (missense) that affect *CPT2* cause the myopathic form of CPT2 deficiency. In individuals of European descent, the most frequent (affecting 60%) results in the replacement of serine with leucine at position 113 (c.338C>T).

Isolated LCHAD deficiency is associated with a homozygous *HADHA* c.1528G>C mutation in most individuals of European descent.

TFP/MTP deficiency due to complete or partial deficiency of all three enzymes (LCEH, LCHAD, LCKAT; page 16) is typically associated with a *HADHA* c.1528G>C (p.Glu510Gln) mutation affecting one allele and an allele carrying a different mutation at the same gene

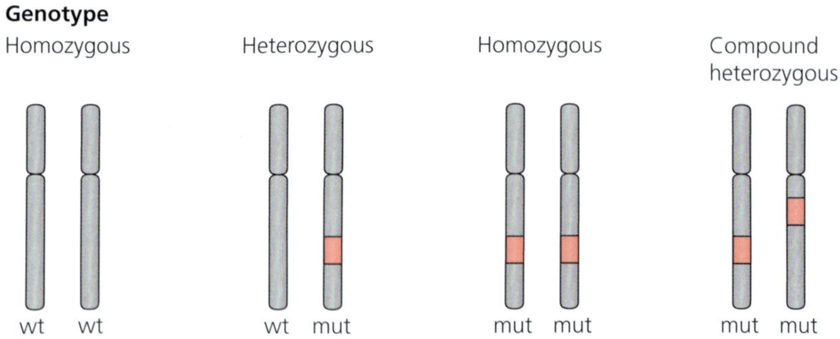

Figure 2.1 The arrangement of mutations in different genotypes. In individuals with a compound heterozygous genotype, two alleles have different recessive mutations at the same locus.

locus on the other chromosome (that is, most patients are compound heterozygotes, Figure 2.1).

A unique polymorphism of the *CPT1A* gene, c.1436C>T (p.Pro479Leu), is associated with decreased enzymatic activity and impaired fasting ketogenesis, which can lead to hypoketotic hypoglycemia in young children. This polymorphism is particularly prevalent among the Canadian and Greenland Inuit and some Alaska Native populations.[10]

Key points – epidemiology and genetics

- Some FAODs have a wide range of clinical presentations, with phenotypic diversity reflecting interactions between genetic and environmental factors.
- The lack of clear association between genotype and clinical symptoms makes clinical management complex.
- The incidence of individual FAODs is difficult to estimate. Newborn screening programs have led to an increase in prevalence of the conditions in some countries.

References

1. Lindner M, Hoffmann GF, Matern D. Newborn screening for disorders of fatty-acid oxidation: experience and recommendations from an expert meeting. *J Inherit Metab Dis* 2010;33:521–6.

2. Leslie ND, Valencia CA, Strauss AW et al. Very long-chain acyl-coenzyme A dehydrogenase deficiency. 2009 (updated 2019). In: Adam MP, Ardinger HH, Pagon RA et al, eds. *GeneReviews®*. University of Washington, 1993–2020. www.ncbi.nlm.nih.gov/books/NBK6816/, last accessed 15 September 2020.

3. Orphanet. Long chain 3-hydroxyacyl-CoA dehydrogenase deficiency. www.orpha.net/consor/cgi-bin/OC_Exp.php?lng=EN&Expert=5, last accessed 15 September 2020.

4. Vockley J. Long-chain fatty acid oxidation disorders and current management strategies. *Am J Manag Care* 2020;26(suppl):S147–54.

5. Bennett MJ, Rinaldo P, Strauss AW. Inborn errors of mitochondrial fatty acid oxidation. *Crit Rev Clin Lab Sci* 2000;37:1–44.

6. Spiekerkoetter U, Mayatepek E. Update on mitochondrial fatty acid oxidation disorders. *J Inherit Metab Dis* 2010;33:467–8.

7. Wanders RJ. Functions and dysfunctions of peroxisomes in fatty acid alpha- and beta-oxidation. New insights. *Adv Exp Med Biol* 1999;466:283–99.

8. Wanders RJ, Komen J, Kemp S. Fatty acid omega-oxidation as a rescue pathway for fatty acid oxidation disorders in humans. *FEBS J* 2011;278:182–94.

9. Spiekerkoetter U, Bennett MJ, Ben-Zeev B et al. Peripheral neuropathy, episodic myoglobinuria, and respiratory failure in deficiency of the mitochondrial trifunctional protein. *Muscle Nerve* 2004;29:66–72.

10. Gillingham MB, Hirschfeld M, Lowe S et al. Impaired fasting tolerance among Alaska native children with a common carnitine palmitoyltransferase 1A sequence variant. *Mol Genet Metab* 2011;104:261–4.

3 Clinical presentation

General symptoms

Many of the most common clinical manifestations of long-chain (LC)-FAODs are shared by all of the individual disorders in the group (Figure 3.1). In addition, there are two important clinical findings that are typically observed only in LCHAD and TFP deficiency, namely peripheral neuropathy and retinopathy.

All of the LC-FAODs exhibit a spectrum of clinical severity, and age of onset can be any time from the immediate neonatal period through adult life. In addition, the phenotype in an individual patient often changes as a function of age. Symptoms such as hypoglycemia and hepatic dysfunction are most common in infants and young children while, in adolescents and adults, the phenotype is often dominated by skeletal myopathy with recurrent rhabdomyolysis and chronic exercise intolerance. Cardiomyopathy, either hypertrophic or dilated, can occur at any age but is most severe in infants and children and may resolve as patients get older. Pericardial effusions may be observed.

Severely affected infants can present in the immediate neonatal period with a severe metabolic crisis, characterized by hypoglycemia, hyperammonemia, hepatic dysfunction, muscle weakness, respiratory distress and seizures with encephalopathy. The conditions most likely to present in this severe fashion are CACT deficiency and the severe form of CPT2 deficiency.

The mortality rate in patients with this severe neonatal presentation is very high.[1] The severe form of CPT2 deficiency may be accompanied by structural malformations such as cystic renal dysplasia, neuronal migration defects of the brain and dysmorphic facial features.[2]

Other LC-FAODs may occasionally present in the neonatal period with less overwhelming symptoms and a greater likelihood of long-term survival.

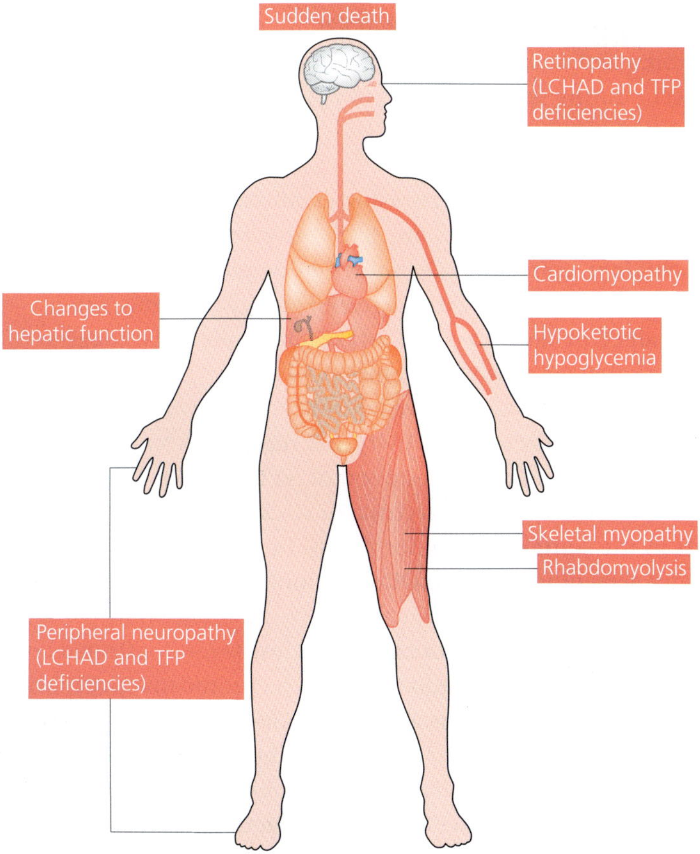

Figure 3.1 Symptoms of LC-FAODs (general and for LCHAD and TFP deficiencies).

Beyond the neonatal period, individuals often present with symptoms of a mild intercurrent illness followed by much more severe signs of illness than would be anticipated.[3] They may present with profound lethargy or coma from hypoglycemia, hypotonia or recurrent vomiting or with respiratory distress and/or circulatory collapse related to cardiac dysfunction or arrhythmias. Hepatomegaly may be present.

Growth retardation occurs with increased frequency, though ultimate stature is typically normal. While intellectual disability is not an intrinsic feature of most LC-FAODs, motor delay related to hypotonia and muscle weakness is not uncommon and brain damage can occur during severe episodes of hypoglycemia or hepatic encephalopathy.

Typical course. LC-FAODs typically exhibit an episodic course, with individuals being asymptomatic or stable between episodes.

In children, episodes of decompensation are typically triggered by intercurrent illnesses with increased energy demands, often accompanied by decreased oral intake. Other potential triggers include prolonged fasting and emotional stress.

Common symptoms observed during acute decompensation include lethargy, decreased activity and recurrent vomiting. Sudden death may be the first manifestation of an LC-FAOD. This is likely attributable either to hypoglycemia or to cardiac arrhythmia and often occurs in the context of a minor illness. In those countries with newborn screening for LC-FAODs, the incidence of sudden death has been significantly reduced.

As patients get older, those who are most severely affected and presented earlier in childhood may have a chronic myopathy with muscle weakness, hypotonia and exercise intolerance, punctuated by episodes of rhabdomyolysis characterized by muscle pain and dark or cola-colored urine. In addition to intercurrent illnesses, such episodes may be precipitated by excessive physical activity.

Patients with a milder disorder, such as the common late-onset forms of CPT2 or VLCAD deficiency, may present for the first time in adolescence or adult life with acute rhabdomyolysis after intense exercise. With muscle cell breakdown, myoglobin is released and can precipitate in the renal tubules, causing acute renal failure. In addition to elevated creatine kinase (CK) levels, patients experiencing rhabdomyolysis may exhibit hyperkalemia and its complications (Table 3.1).

Abnormal laboratory findings in LC-FAODs may include:

- hypoketotic hypoglycemia
- elevated ammonia and transaminases
- elevated CK.

TABLE 3.1

Signs and symptoms of rhabdomyolysis

- Fever, confusion, loss of consciousness
- Abnormal or irregular heartbeat
- Dark-colored urine or low volumes of urine
- Trouble moving items or lifting objects
- Nausea and vomiting
- Muscle swelling
- Muscle weakness or fatigue in legs
- High levels of potassium in bloodstream
- General feeling of malaise, fatigue or illness

CK typically rises during an episode of metabolic decompensation. During acute episodes of rhabdomyolysis, it may be extremely elevated. Some individuals, particularly older patients with severe defects, have chronic elevations of CK. During a significant episode of rhabdomyolysis, the urine will test positive on dipstick for occult blood because of the presence of myoglobin. Serum potassium may be elevated and, if renal function is compromised, blood urea nitrogen and creatinine may be elevated.

Symptoms of specific LC-FAODs

Carnitine transporter deficiency (CTD; also referred to as carnitine uptake defect [CUD], and systemic carnitine deficiency). This disorder results in a defect in the transport of carnitine, primarily derived from the diet, across plasma membranes into cells and results in excess carnitine loss in the urine.

As carnitine is essential to the import of fatty acids into the mitochondria, the consequence of this defect is impairment of fatty acid oxidation. Some patients with CTD exhibit the typical manifestations of LC-FAOD, including hypoglycemia, hepatic dysfunction and encephalopathy, while others have isolated cardiomyopathy with increased risk of arrhythmias and sudden death.[4]

A significant number of people with CTD may remain asymptomatic for long periods of time, possibly for life. This has been recognized since newborn screening for the condition began.

Low levels of free carnitine (C0) in a newborn infant may reflect maternal carnitine deficiency, which may be dietary in some instances but may also lead to the diagnosis of CTD in the mother. These mothers are often asymptomatic or report non-specific symptoms of fatigue and exercise intolerance that have never led to the consideration of an inherited metabolic disorder. Carnitine deficiency is typically severe, even in those individuals reporting no symptoms.

CACT deficiency prevents LCFAs from being transported from the cytosol of the cell into the intramitochondrial space for oxidation and energy production. This rare disorder is typically severe, with onset of symptoms in the neonatal period.[1]

Clinical findings include respiratory distress, cardiomyopathy, muscle weakness, seizures, hepatomegaly, hypoketotic hypoglycemia and hyperammonemia. There is a high rate of mortality with this neonatal presentation, but a subset of individuals have a somewhat milder phenotype or present later in life. As surviving individuals grow older, they begin to experience episodes of rhabdomyolysis.

CPT1A deficiency. The early-onset form of CPT1A deficiency presents with episodes of acute liver failure and hepatic encephalopathy, accompanied by hypoketotic hypoglycemia and hyperammonemia, which are typically triggered by intercurrent illnesses.[5] Hepatomegaly is often present.

Individuals with milder defects may present later in adolescence or adult life with episodes of rhabdomyolysis associated with muscle pain and weakness. In contrast to all other LC-FAODs, cardiac manifestations are rare in CPT1A deficiency.

CPT2 deficiency. Three clinical subtypes of CPT2 deficiency are recognized, though individuals may have an intermediate phenotype.

The first subtype is the neonatal lethal form, which is associated with hepatic and cardiac dysfunction, encephalopathy, seizures, hypotonia and muscle weakness, hypoglycemia and hyperammonemia. Affected infants often also have structural malformations, such as cystic renal dysplasia, neuronal migration defects of the brain and dysmorphic facial features. Survival is rare.

The infantile form presents slightly later but usually within the first year of life. The symptoms, which are typical of LC-FAOD, include liver dysfunction, cardiomyopathy, skeletal myopathy and hypoglycemia.

Individuals with the common later-onset myopathic form of the disorder exhibit episodes of muscle weakness and pain due to rhabdomyolysis. Typically, between attacks they are completely normal with no hypotonia or muscle weakness detectable.[6] Indeed, some have become serious athletes.

Onset of symptoms commonly occurs in childhood, even in the late-onset form of the disorder, but diagnosis is often delayed for many years if episodes are not severe and are self-resolving with rest. Infrequently, affected individuals do not experience any symptoms until adult life; some may remain largely asymptomatic if they avoid vigorous exercise, which is the most common precipitating factor. Other triggers include infection, fasting or occasionally general anesthesia, extreme cold or excessive fatigue.

VLCAD deficiency is a highly variable disorder.[7] In its severe form, patients exhibit all of the characteristic features of an LC-FAOD from early infancy. Individuals with milder defects present later in childhood or adolescence with recurrent rhabdomyolysis and exercise intolerance.

Symptoms such as hepatic dysfunction, hypoglycemia and cardiomyopathy predominate in the severely affected patients in the early years of life. Over time, however, the phenotype evolves, and these patients also primarily exhibit skeletal myopathy and recurrent rhabdomyolysis in adult life.

It is possible that some individuals with VLCAD deficiency remain asymptomatic. Of patients detected by newborn screening, a significant fraction do not have symptoms in early childhood and have remained asymptomatic into their teens. While further follow-up may reveal symptoms later in life, it is clear that the mild form of the disorder is the most common subtype.

LCHAD and TFP deficiencies are closely related disorders that are clinically indistinguishable. Most individuals present in infancy or early childhood with the typical manifestations of an LC-FAOD, including hepatic dysfunction, hypoglycemia, cardiomyopathy and sudden death. Those individuals who survive exhibit an evolving phenotype, with skeletal myopathy, recurrent rhabdomyolysis and exercise intolerance developing over time. In addition, patients with this disorder have the unique features of peripheral sensorimotor neuropathy, resulting in loss of deep tendon reflexes early in childhood,[8] and pigmentary retinopathy with progressive but variable visual loss.[9]

Key points – clinical presentation

- Common symptoms of LC-FAODs include hypoglycemia, hepatic dysfunction, cardiomyopathy, skeletal myopathy and rhabdomyolysis.
- Peripheral neuropathy and retinopathy occur in LCHAD deficiency and TFP deficiency.
- Hypoglycemia and hepatic dysfunction are primarily observed in young children, while rhabdomyolysis and exercise intolerance dominate the phenotype in adolescents and adults.
- Acute episodes of decompensation in LC-FAODs are most often precipitated by intercurrent illnesses.

References

1. Wilcken B. Fatty acid oxidation disorders: outcome and long-term prognosis. *J Inherit Metab Dis* 2010;33:501–6.

2. Boemer F, Deberq M, Schoos R et al. Diagnostic pitfall in antenatal manifestations of CPTII deficiency. *Clin Genet* 2016;89:193–7.

3. Knottnerus SJG, Bleeker JC, Wust RCI et al. Disorders of mitochondrial long-chain fatty acid oxidation and the carnitine shuttle. *Rev Endocr Metab Disord* 2018; 19:93–106.

4. El-Hattab AW, Scaglia F. Disorders of carnitine biosynthesis and transport. *Mol Genet Metab* 2015; 116:107–12.

5. Bonnefont JP, Djouadi F, Prip-Buus C et al. Carnitine palmitoyltransferases 1 and 2: biochemical, molecular and medical aspects. *Mol Aspects Med* 2004; 25:495–520.

6. Deschauer M, Wieser T, Zierz S. Muscle carnitine palmitoyltransferase II deficiency: clinical and molecular genetic features and diagnostic aspects. *Arch Neurol* 2005;62:37–41.

7. Pena LD, van Calcar SC, Hansen J et al. Outcomes and genotype-phenotype correlations in 52 individuals with VLCAD deficiency diagnosed by newborn screening and enrolled in the IBEM-IS database. *Mol Genet Metab* 2016;118:272–81.

8. Olpin SE, Clark S, Andresen BS et al. Biochemical, clinical and molecular findings in LCHAD and general mitochondrial trifunctional protein deficiency. *J Inherit Metab Dis* 2005;28:533–44.

9. Fletcher AL, Pennesi ME, Harding CO et al. Observations regarding retinopathy in mitochondrial trifunctional protein deficiencies. *Mol Genet Metab* 2012; 106:18–24.

4 Diagnosis

Individuals with an LC-FAOD may be diagnosed after clinical presentation or after newborn screening while asymptomatic.

Newborn screening

Newborn screening for LC-FAODs is conducted by analysis of acylcarnitines in the dried blood spot obtained from a baby during the first few days of life. Mortality resulting from FAODs has been significantly reduced in countries in which this is available.[1,2]

Following a positive newborn screen for one of these conditions, diagnostic testing must be performed. For most disorders this includes a plasma acylcarnitine profile and urine organic acid analysis. Measurement of free and total carnitine levels is essential when the newborn screen shows findings suggestive of carnitine uptake defect.

It is important to note that both the plasma acylcarnitine profile and urine organic acids are most likely to yield abnormal results when a patient is acutely symptomatic or following fasting. Therefore, normal results of these tests following a positive newborn screen do not rule out the diagnosis of an LC-FAOD.

While patients with the most severe defects will typically have an abnormal acylcarnitine profile regardless of when it is obtained, individuals with milder defects may exhibit abnormalities only when stressed. Newborn screening specimens are typically obtained shortly after the stress of labor and delivery, when feeding may not yet be well established. In contrast, by the time of follow-up testing, infants are typically feeding frequently so are essentially always in a fed state.

Normalization of the acylcarnitine profile has been most commonly observed in infants with a positive newborn screen for VLCAD and LCHAD/TFP deficiencies. These infants should have either some assessment of enzyme activity or molecular testing of the relevant gene or genes, regardless of the biochemical test results.

In some countries, enzyme assays can be performed on blood samples or cultured fibroblasts obtained from a skin biopsy. In other circumstances, indirect evidence of impaired β-oxidation can be obtained by incubating fibroblasts with ^{13}C-labeled or unlabeled palmitate and carnitine, with subsequent acylcarnitine profiling of the cells. This type of study is often referred to as an in-vitro probe study.

Specific algorithms for follow-up of an abnormal newborn screen for each of the LC-FAODs can be found on the website of the American College of Medical Genetics and Genomics (www.acmg.net) under newborn screening and the steps are summarized, with additional notes from the authors, in Table 4.1.

Clinical presentation

If an individual presents with symptoms suggestive of an LC-FAOD, the following studies should be obtained:

- plasma free and total carnitine levels
- plasma acylcarnitine profile
- urine organic acids.

There are characteristic acylcarnitine abnormalities associated with the various disorders (Table 4.2). The acylcarnitine profile is reliably abnormal in all patients only during an acute episode of decompensation and may normalize in some individuals when they are well. Therefore, if a person is seen for evaluation after recovery from the initial episode that prompted concern, it is important that the test be repeated when the patient again develops symptoms.

Urine organic acids are often abnormal during acute episodes but are commonly normal during other times. For some of the disorders, the characteristic findings are those of dicarboxylic aciduria, which are non-specific. In the case of LCHAD/TFP deficiencies, the organic acid abnormalities are more characteristic but do not differentiate between the two conditions.

A disorder that presents with acute episodes of metabolic decompensation and findings very similar to those observed in classic LC-FAOD is TANGO2 encephalopathy with arrhythmias.[3] Ventricular arrhythmias are particularly prominent in this disorder during acute illness. If an individual is suspected of having an LC-FAOD but diagnostic testing is unrevealing, this disorder should

TABLE 4.1

Follow-up for abnormal newborn screening

Finding	Assay	Result	Optional tests to confirm
Decreased C0	Free and total carnitine in plasma and urine*	Plasma C0: low	Transporter assay
Other ACs relatively low		Plasma total carnitine: normal/low	*OCTN2* (*SLC22A5*) genetic testing
		Carnitine transporter deficiency	
Elevated/normal C0	Plasma carnitine	Plasma C0: high	CPT1 assay
Elevated C0/C16 + C18	Plasma AC	Plasma AC: normal, or	*CPT1A* gene analysis
		Long-chain AC: low	
		CPT1 deficiency	
Elevated C16 and/ or C18:1	1 Plasma AC	CPT2/CACT profile	
		Go to 2	
	2 Fibroblast culture		
	CPT2 assay	Positive	*CPT2* gene analysis†
		CPT2 deficiency	
	CACT assay	Positive	
		CACT deficiency	

Elevated C16-OH ± C18:1-OH and other long-chain ACs	1 Plasma AC Urine OA	Plasma AC: LCHAD/TFP profile Urine OA: normal or LCHAD/TFP profile **LCHAD/TFP deficiency‡** *If results normal, go to 2*	LCHAD/TFP enzyme assays LCHAD/TFP gene(s) analysis
	2 In vitro FAO assay (fibroblasts/ lymphoblasts)	LCHAD/TFP profile **LCHAD/TFP deficiency**	
Elevation of C8 Lesser elevations of C6 and C10	Plasma AC Urine OA Urine AG	Plasma AC (C8): high Urine OA: normal/high dicarboxylic acids Urine AG: high hexanoylglycine **MCAD deficiency**	*MCAD* (*ACADM*) gene sequencing
C4-OH elevated	Plasma AC Urine OA Plasma insulin	Plasma C4-OH: high Urine OA: OH-DCA Plasma insulin: high/normal **HADH deficiency§**	*HADH* gene sequencing

(CONTINUED)

TABLE 4.1 (CONTINUED)

Follow-up for abnormal newborn screening

Finding	Assay	Result	Optional tests to confirm
Elevated C4 and C5 ± other ACs	Plasma AC	Plasma AC: MADD/GA2 profile	ETF/ETF-QO assay
	Urine OA	Urine OA: MADD/GA2 profile	ETF/ETF-QO gene sequencing
	Urine AG	Urine AG: MADD/GA2 profile	
		MADD/GA2	
		Plasma AC: C4 ± C5	*ETHE1* gene sequencing
		Urine OA: EE/IVG	
		Urine AG: EE + IVG	
		Ethylmalonic encephalopathy 1	
		Plasma AC: normal	ETF/ETF-QO assay
		Urine OA: normal	ETF/ETF-QO gene sequencing
		Urine AG: normal	
		False positive (normal) or mild MADD/GA2	

Elevation of C14:1 ± 1 other long-chain AC	Plasma AC, quantitative	Plasma AC: VLCAD profile **VLCAD deficiency‡**	*VLCAD* (*ACADVL*) gene sequencing FAO probe assay (fibroblast culture)
			FAO: C12<C14<C16 **Severe VLCAD deficiency**
			FAO: C10<C12>C14 **Mild VLCAD deficiency**

Based on recommendations from the American College of Medical Genetics and Genomics (www.acmg.net).
Where an older gene symbol is shown, the up-to-date symbol is shown in parentheses.
*Maternal plasma free and total carnitine should also be measured. Mild deficiencies in mother and infant may result from dietary carnitine deficiency.
†This can be done on blood to confirm diagnosis if fibroblast culture not obtained.
‡The plasma AC profile may normalize in the fed state following a positive newborn screen, particularly in mild cases. A normal AC profile should not be taken as evidence to exclude the diagnosis. Enzyme assay or molecular testing should be done in every case.
§Also known as M/SCHAD deficiency. If results are normal, consult a metabolic disease specialist, who may consider enzyme assays in fibroblasts and/or *HADH* mutation analysis.
AC, acylcarnitine; AG, acylglycine; C4-OH, 3-hydroxybutyrylcarnitine; C16-OH, 3-hydroxypalmitoylcarnitine; C18:1-OH, 3-hydroxyoleoylcarnitine; DCA, dicarboxylic acid; EE, ethylmalonic encephalopathy 1; ETF(-QO), electron transfer flavoprotein (dehydrogenase); FAO, fatty acid oxidation; GA2, glutaric aciduria type 2; IVG, isovaleryl glycine; MADD, multiple acyl-CoA dehydrogenase deficiency; OA, organic acid; SCHAD, short-chain 3-hydroxyacyl-CoA dehydrogenase.

TABLE 4.2

Characteristic acylcarnitine abnormalities in LC-FAOD

Disorder	Abnormalities
CTD	↓C0
CPT1 deficiency	↑C0, ↓C2, ↑C0/C16 + C18
CACT deficiency	↑C16, ↑C18, ↑C18:1, ↑C18:2
CPT2 deficiency	↑C16, ↑C18, ↑C18:1, ↑C18:2
VLCAD deficiency	↑C12, ↑C14, ↑C14:1, ↑C16, ↑C18
LCHAD, TFP deficiency	↑C14-OH, ↑C16, ↑C16-OH, ↑C18-OH, ↑C18:1-OH

be considered. It is confirmed by the demonstration of biallelic mutations in *TANGO2*.

Plasma free carnitine, acylcarnitines and total carnitine levels are typically all very low in patients with carnitine uptake disorder. Patients with CPT1A deficiency have elevated total carnitine levels. Carnitine levels are variable in the other disorders, but secondary carnitine deficiency is not uncommon. There is often an increase in the ratio of acylcarnitines to free carnitine, and the free carnitine level may be abnormally low.

Some patients who experience recurrent rhabdomyolysis as their presenting symptom may have a muscle biopsy done before undergoing biochemical testing for an LC-FAOD. While this can be avoided in individuals with an LC-FAOD if the appropriate metabolic testing is obtained during the acute episode, there are some other metabolic disorders that can only be accurately diagnosed in this way. If muscle biopsy is done, typically the tissue is sent for a panel of either enzymatic tests or molecular tests for conditions leading to rhabdomyolysis. This should lead to the diagnosis of VLCAD or CPT2 deficiency, the two forms of LC-FAOD most likely to present in this way. Other disorders may be included depending on the testing laboratory.

Conditions in the differential diagnosis of recurrent rhabdomyolysis include McArdle disease and some primary myopathies. A single episode of rhabdomyolysis can have a non-genetic etiology, such as crush injury, electrical shock, drug toxicity, heat stroke, extreme muscle strain or infection.

Postmortem diagnosis

If a patient experiences sudden death, testing can be performed postmortem. One large series of 418 cases of sudden death in the first year of life revealed that 5–8% were the result of FAODs.[4] This was based on a combination of postmortem analyses on the deceased infants and studies of surviving siblings.

The possibility of an FAOD is suggested by the presence of microvesicular steatosis in the liver. It is strengthened if fat deposition is also noted in other tissues, such as myocardium, skeletal muscle and kidney. If a frozen plasma sample is available from a person who has died suddenly with these findings, an acylcarnitine profile should be obtained. If frozen unfixed tissue is available, enzymatic testing or acylcarnitine profiling of liver tissue may be possible.

Molecular testing can be performed on frozen tissue and often also on tissue obtained from a paraffin block. If none of these is possible, sequencing of the FAOD genes can be performed on samples from the parents to determine if both are carriers of a detectable mutation in one of the relevant genes.

Key points – diagnosis

- If a patient presents with clinical findings suggestive of an LC-FAOD, obtain: plasma free and total carnitine levels; plasma acylcarnitine profile; and urine organic acids.
- Urine organic acids and the plasma acylcarnitine profile may be normal when the patient is well. If a diagnosis is not established, testing should be repeated during an acute episode.
- After a positive newborn screen for VLCAD or LCHAD/TFP deficiency, the acylcarnitine profile may normalize. Molecular testing is essential to rule out these diagnoses.
- A condition that is very similar clinically to LC-FAOD is *TANGO2*-related metabolic encephalopathy. If an LC-FAOD is suspected but diagnostic testing is unrevealing, this disorder should be considered.

References

1. Spiekerkoetter U. Mitochondrial fatty acid oxidation disorders: clinical presentation of long-chain fatty acid oxidation defects before and after newborn screening. *J Inherit Metab Dis* 2010:33:527–32.

2. Wilcken B. Fatty acid oxidation disorders: outcome and long-term prognosis. *J Inherit Metab Dis* 2010:33:501–6.

3. Dines JN, Golden-Grant K, LaCroix A et al. TANGO2: expanding the clinical phenotype and spectrum of pathogenic variants. *Genet Med* 2019:21:601–7.

4. Boles RG, Buck EA, Blitzer MG et al. Retrospective biochemical screening of fatty acid oxidation disorders in postmortem livers of 418 cases of sudden death in the first year of life. *J Pediatr* 1998:132:924–33.

5 Genetic counseling, newborn screening and patient support

Pattern of inheritance

All LC-FAODs are inherited in an autosomal recessive pattern. Therefore, a couple who have had one affected child face a risk of 25%, or one in four, in any future pregnancy of having another affected child (Figure 5.1).

While adult patients with an LC-FAOD will always transmit the gene for their disorder to a child, there is a relatively low risk that a child will be affected as both parents must transmit the recessive gene to the child for this to occur.

Siblings of individuals with an LC-FAOD have a risk of two in three of carrying the recessive gene (see Figure 5.1) but again, the risk of having an affected child is low as the partner would also need to be a carrier.

Testing

Carrier testing is available for couples with a family history of an LC-FAOD (for example, where one partner has an LC-FAOD or an affected sibling) who want to further define their risk. For relatives of affected patients in whom the causative mutations are known, testing can be done for the presence of those specific mutations. In the case of unrelated partners, gene sequencing is required.

Prenatal diagnosis can be achieved by chorionic villus sampling in the first trimester or amniocentesis in the second trimester and molecular testing on the fetal cells. Preimplantation genetic diagnosis is also possible if both causative mutations have been identified in the index patient and the couple is willing to undergo in-vitro fertilization.

Newborn testing. ***At-risk infant.*** When no prenatal diagnosis is performed in a pregnancy known to be at risk for an LC-FAOD, the newborn should be tested immediately after birth. All families with a new diagnosis of an LC-FAOD should be referred to a genetic counselor

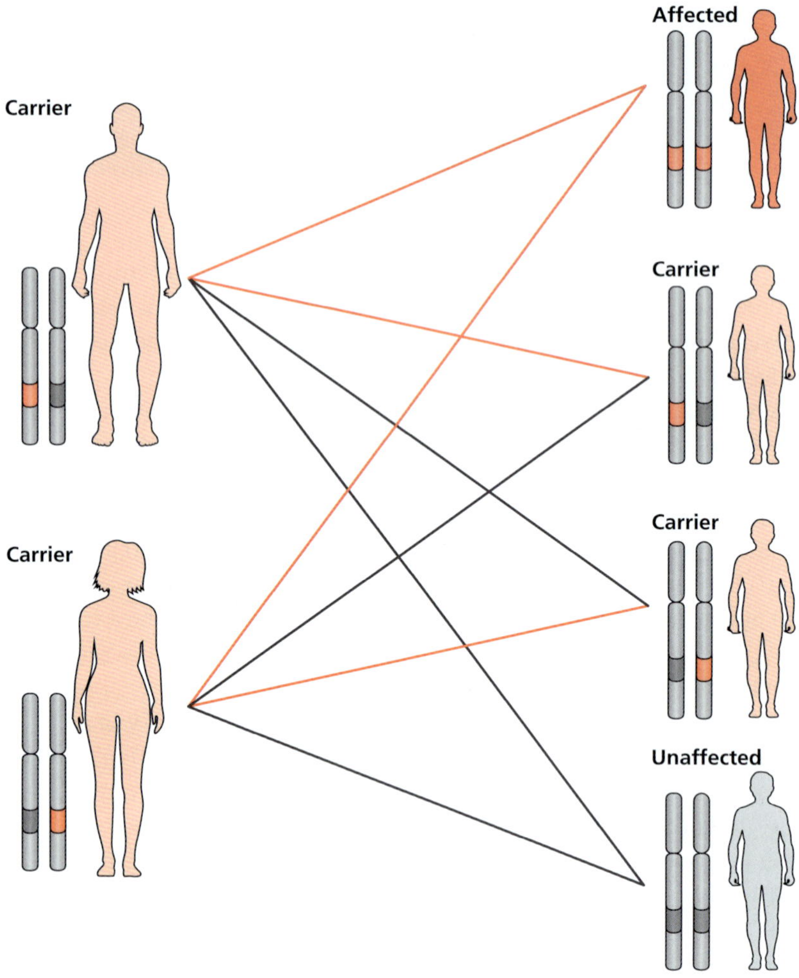

Figure 5.1 The risk of a child being affected if both parents have an autosomal recessive gene for a specific LC-FAOD is 25%.

to discuss the pattern of inheritance, reproductive risks and options for addressing those risks, as well as the emotional impact of the diagnosis of a potentially life-threatening genetic disorder.

Pregnancy complications linked to LC-FAODs. When the fetus is affected, some of the LC-FAODs are associated with an increased risk of intrauterine growth restriction, prematurity and pregnancy complications, such as severe preeclampsia, acute fatty liver of pregnancy and the hemolysis, elevated liver enzymes and low platelets (HELLP) syndrome. This is particularly true when the fetus is affected with LCHAD or TFP deficiency,[1] but an association has also been reported in CPT1A deficiency. If there is no universal newborn screening for LC-FAODs after birth these complications should prompt consideration that the newborn may be affected, even when there is no history of an LC-FAOD in the family.

Screening

Newborn screening for LC-FAODs is performed routinely in some countries around the world. The dried blood spot obtained from the infant in the first few days of life is analyzed for acylcarnitines. Follow-up biochemical testing after a positive newborn screen can be normal, even in an affected infant. Therefore, molecular testing, enzyme assay or some other functional assessment of LCFA oxidation should be performed to avoid missing an affected infant.

If an infant or child presents with findings suggestive of an LC-FAOD, diagnostic testing should be pursued even if there was a normal result on newborn screening. Occasional cases, particularly those with milder defects, will be missed by newborn screening even under optimal conditions.

Counseling

Parents and patients of all ages should receive regular counseling and education regarding their diagnosis. In particular, they should be educated regarding triggers of acute decompensation so that these may be avoided whenever possible.

Fasting avoidance. Fasting is clearly the trigger that is most easily avoided. From birth until 6 months of age, affected infants should be fed every 3–4 hours. By 6 months of age, the period between feedings during the night can be extended to 6 hours and this can gradually increase until 1 year of age, at which time infants, when well, should be able to sleep for up to 10–12 hours at night without feeding.

Illness. During respiratory illnesses or when fever is present, parents should be instructed to revert to feeding breast milk, infant formula or

TABLE 5.1

Symptoms of hypoglycemia and metabolic decompensation for discussion with families

- Lethargy
- Difficulty being aroused from sleep
- Poor feeding – disinterest in sucking, falling asleep early in a feeding
- Recurrent vomiting

a glucose-containing beverage every 3–4 hours. Families should be acquainted with the symptoms of hypoglycemia and metabolic decompensation (Table 5.1) and should be instructed to seek medical care early in the course of any intercurrent illness.

Parents should not rely on home glucose monitoring to alert them to when the child needs medical care. If the child has symptoms of lethargy, recurrent vomiting or poor oral intake, medical evaluation should occur, regardless of whether the blood glucose is low.

If an individual with an LC-FAOD is unable to tolerate oral feeding, intravenous glucose may be necessary to avoid the catabolic stress that precipitates acute decompensation.

Exercise and physical activity. Skeletal myopathy becomes the predominant problem for most patients as they get older. Individuals should be counseled about appropriate levels of exercise and physical activity. In addition, they should be instructed that muscle pain, increased or new-onset weakness and dark urine are all signs of rhabdomyolysis, which should prompt communication with the medical provider.

Identification. All patients should be provided with an emergency letter that details their diagnosis, as well as steps to be taken in the case of acute symptoms prompting presentation to an emergency facility. Contact information for the medical care team familiar with the patient should be included. Patients should be instructed to show this letter at the time of any visit for urgent or emergency care.

Patient support. There are a number of professional organizations and advocacy groups that can be useful sources of information and support for families of individuals with an LC-FAOD. Some of these are listed in the Useful resources section (page 46).

Key points – genetic counseling, newborn screening and patient support

- Parents or patients with a newly diagnosed LC-FAOD should be referred for genetic counseling to discuss the inheritance of the disorder and the implications for their family.
- Regular patient and parent education is an essential component of care of individuals with an LC-FAOD.
- Patients should be counseled regularly on how to avoid triggers of acute metabolic decompensation.

Reference

1. Shekhawat PS, Matern D, Strauss AW. Fetal fatty acid oxidation disorders, their effect on maternal health and neonatal outcome: implications of expanded newborn screening on their diagnosis and management. *Pediatr Res* 2005;57:78R–86R.

Useful resources

International Network for Fatty Acid Oxidation Research and Management (INFORM)
A global scientific organization focusing on FAODs and related enzymatic disorders involving the carnitine transport cycle. Professional and patient resources

informnetwork.org

Orphanet
A portal for rare diseases and orphan drugs

www.orphanet.net

USA

FOD Family Support Group
A patient support organization

fodsupport.org

MitoAction
A patient organization that aims to improve the quality of life for children, adults and families living with mitochondrial disease through support, education, outreach, advocacy and clinical research initiatives

www.mitoaction.org

National Organization for Rare Disorders (NORD)
Professional and patient resources

rarediseases.org

Everylife Foundation for Rare Diseases
An organization dedicated to advancing the development of treatments and diagnostic mechanisms for rare diseases through science-driven public policy

everylifefoundation.org

Save Babies Through Screening Foundation
An organization with the goal of ensuring every baby born in the USA is screened successfully, effectively and comprehensively

www.savebabies.org

Canada

MitoCanada
A patient organization that aims to provide diagnosed individuals, their families and caregivers with knowledge and support to improve quality of life while raising public awareness of mitochondrial disease and advancing Canadian research activities

mitocanada.org

UK

British Inherited Metabolic Disease Group (BIMDG)
A group of healthcare professionals dedicated to advancing the education of those involved in caring for and treating people with inherited metabolic diseases, and promoting research into the treatment of these diseases

www.bimdg.org.uk

Metabolic Support UK
A patient organization for inherited metabolic disorders

www.metabolicsupportuk.org

Index